The 30 Day Self-Esteem Journaling Journey

Rhea Hill, MS, LPC, NCC

Copyright © 2021 by Rhea L. Hill

All rights reserved, including the right to reproduce this book or portions thereof in any form whatsoever. For information, address the publisher at:

Blissed Being
1229 E. Pleasant Run Rd.
Ste. 305
Dallas, TX 75115-8621
info@blissedbeing.com

Visit the authors website at:
www.blissedbeing.com
https://www.facebook.com/blissedbeing
https://www.instagram.com/blissedbeing
https://twitter.com/blissedbeing

Printed in the United States of America

First Printing, 2021

ISBN: 978-1-7364637-0-3

"You yourself, as much as anybody in the entire universe, deserve your love and affection."

Buddha

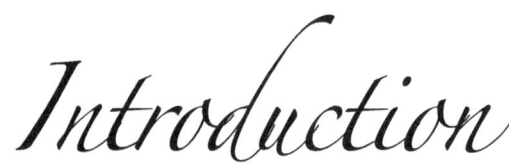

Introduction

Greetings, Blissed Beings, and welcome to The 30-Day Self-Esteem Journaling Journey! Better yet, welcome to securing a heightened awareness of self-esteem. Nurturing your self-esteem for just a few moments of your day can provide you with increased awareness and an assured sense of who you are- live in your purpose. This journal offers writing prompts that encourage exploration and a healthy sense of self. All you have to do is follow the prompts for 30 days without exceptions or excuses; after all, they just get in the way of self-care. Take this opportunity for growth using a meaningful, engaging journal guide to inspire and enhance your very being.

Self-esteem, defined, is confidence and satisfaction in oneself. Understandably this concept is widely used. Esteem is the respect or admiration you hold yourself or someone else.

So, let's open our minds to the notion that self-esteem is a direct experience with our core awareness, which would suggest that self-esteem is beyond our ego. True self-esteem does not feel shame, hubris, or bitterness because the core awareness of being equal to all is inherently accepted.

Consider the book in your hands to be your personal experience and opportunity to connect with your inner self. Your self-reflections will have a meaningful impact on your mental processes. Identify a scheduled time to write and create a consistent routine. Start with small writing time increments, like 10 minutes, and set a timer. You can practice this journaling journey in the morning as a positive start to your day or at night as a time of reflection.

Aspire to designate a quiet space for solace and peace. For example, outdoors in nature or a calm spot in your home- get creative. Prepare with breathing and meditation before each journaling prompt.

Follow this book of journaling prompts daily for the next 30-days consistently, and you'll experience increased awareness and improved self-esteem.

The Attitude of Gratitude

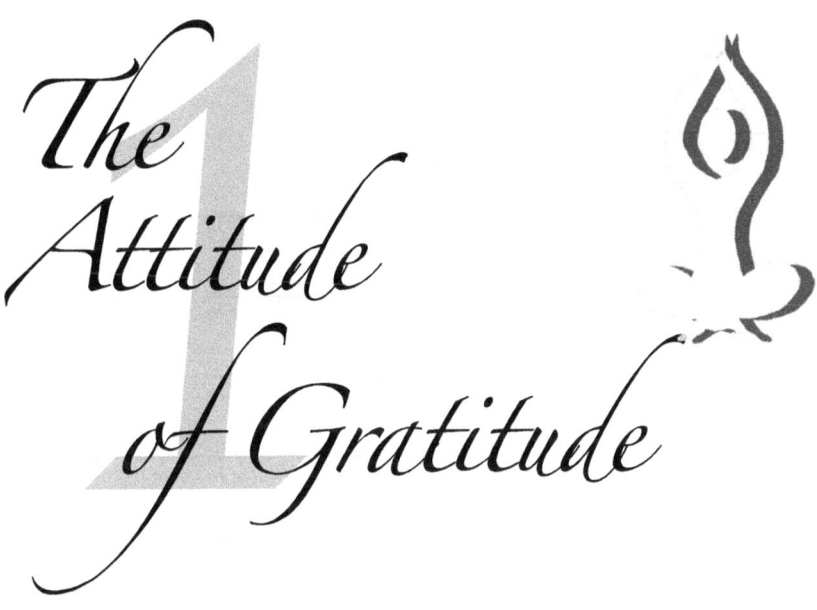

Practicing gratitude will change your focus from negative thoughts to a higher enlightened view of life. Gratitude improves physical and psychological health, enhances your empathy for others, and improves your self-esteem.

Bring your focus to your heart center. Spend some time in solitude and ask yourself, "What are three things that I am grateful for?" How have they benefited you physically, mentally, emotionally, and spiritually? Provide details. When you've completed this journaling entry, concentrate on things you are grateful for throughout your day.

Reflect on The 2 Important People

Wholesome relationships are essential for healthy connections in our lives. Most of us have experienced bonds that have endured pain, and some with sustained fulfillment. Take a moment and reflect on at least one significant person in your life. Write about how the ties with that person have positively transformed you and how you have influenced them.

Unique Qualities

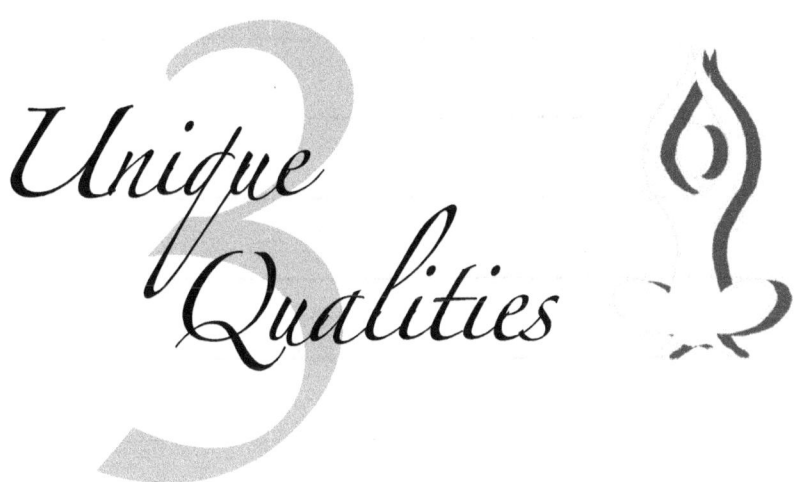

On this lovely day, focus on your unique qualities. Everyone is novel in their own right, and we all have a distinctive gift to give. Focus on your characteristics and talents, identify them, and journal your thoughts and feelings about your attributes.

_____

_____

_____

_____

_____

How can you implement your unique talents in different capacities like home, work, and school?

Positivity Through 4 Challenges

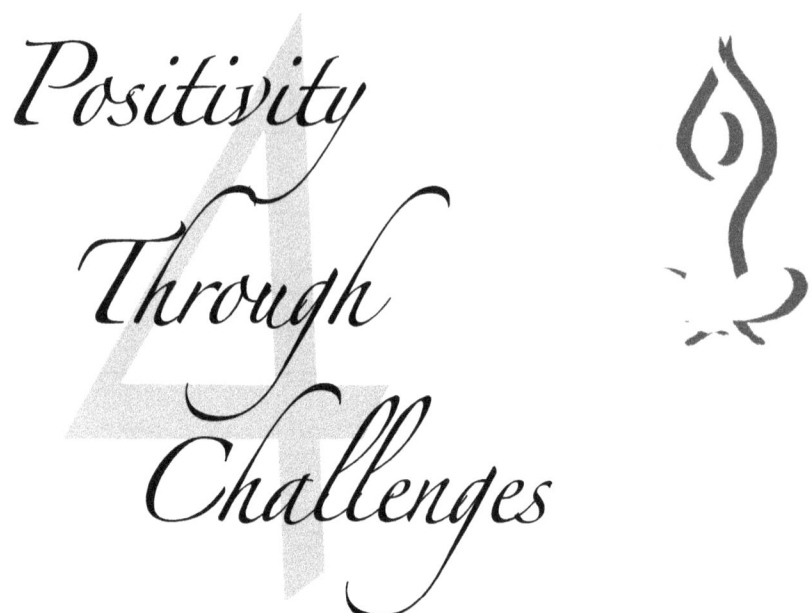

Life brings about many challenges; it is inevitable. Reflect on a struggle that has fostered your personal growth. Write what you feel about the hurdle and how you survived the trial. What did you learn? How do you use your development today?

_____

_____

_____

_____

5 Honor Your Strengths

Recognizing your strengths as gifts contributes to clarity and confidence. When you are clear about your divine empowerments and what you do extraordinarily well, you are in a position to use your inner strengths. Write down at least three strengths with supporting examples of actions, accomplishments, or behaviors that demonstrate each power. Identify how you survived your most notable storm.

Your Gifts Will Return to You

"Give, and you will receive. Your gift will return to you in full-pressed down, shaken together to make room for more, running over, and poured into your lap. The amount you give will determine the amount you get back." Luke 6:38 NLT

Remember the saying, "What you put out is what you get back." What you give is what you receive. For example, if you are seeking acceptance, practice acceptance of others. Suppose you're looking for respect, show and set a standard of reverence for others, and you will receive the same. If more money is what you seek, generate more income, and share with others. In this journal entry, tap into your inner awareness and identify the gifts you can grow.

Reflections

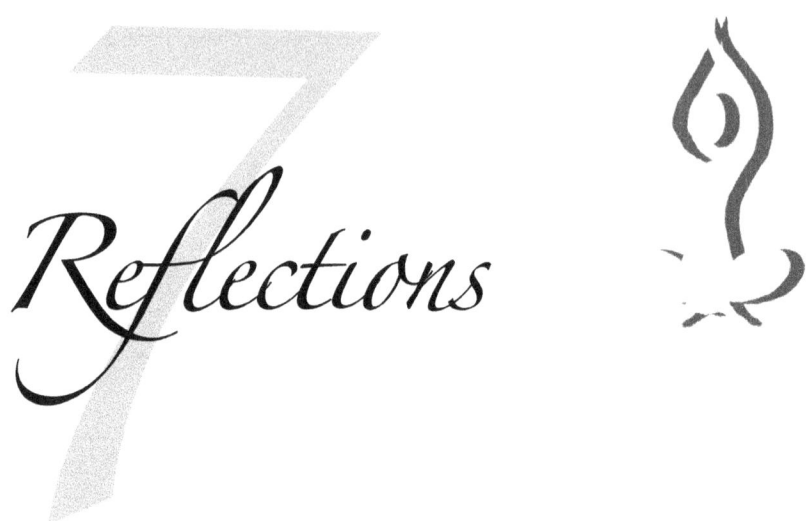

After reading the statement below, envision how you can apply this thought to your relationships and daily interactions, then journal your reflections.

"I am below no one; I am higher than no one. I am equal to all. I am immune to flattery and criticism but receptive to insight. I am free of good and bad opinions. I effectively interact with people without attachment to the outcome."

Build Self-Esteem

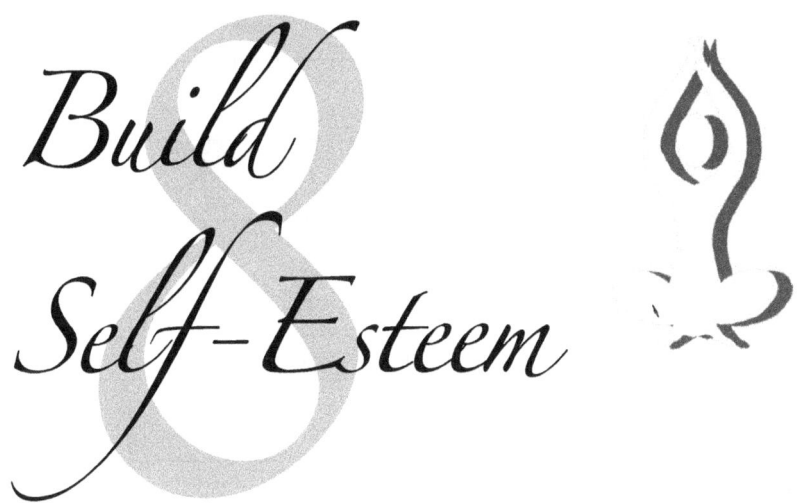

Below are five self-esteem building activities. Please read them and engage in one that resonates with you. Start by journaling how you believe the practice will benefit you, and after you have completed the exercise, journal your observations.

- Practice a random act of kindness.
- Surround yourself with supportive people.
- Demonstrate your unique talents and share them with others.
- Spend time in meditation.
- Exercise

Alternative Perspective

Think about one negative view you have about yourself and write it down. Now, challenge your thought by asking yourself, "Is it fact or opinion? Accurate or inaccurate? Helpful or unhelpful?" Directly change your outlook by practicing a more balanced and realistic perspective. Then, journal an alternative positive belief that will crush your negative perception.

10 Younger Self

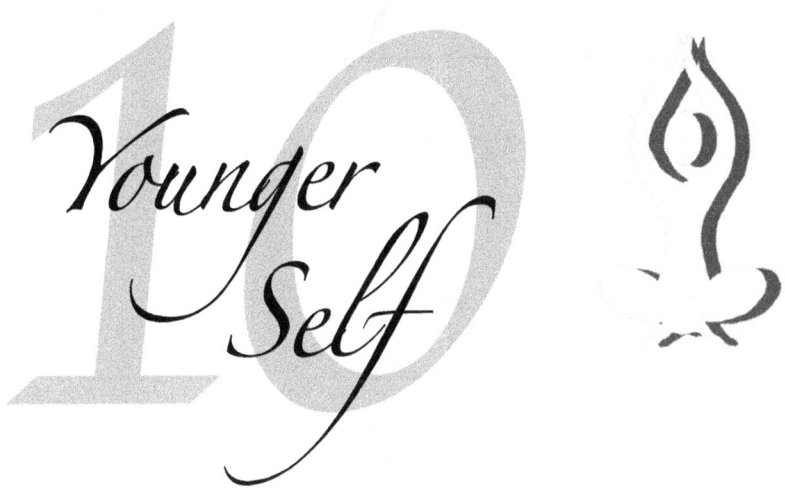

Take a moment and imagine yourself at a younger age. What advice would you give to your younger self? How can you apply this sound advice to yourself today?

_____
_____
_____
_____
_____

The Silver Lining

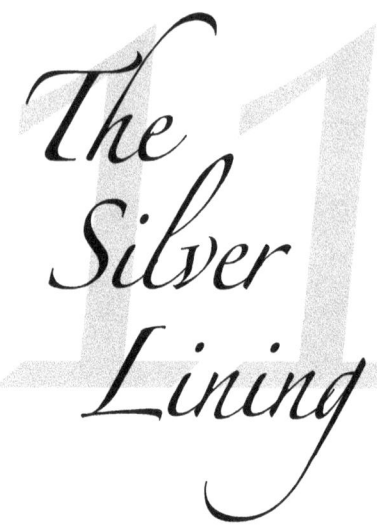
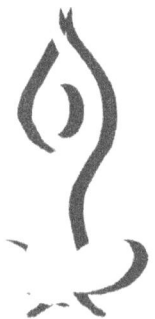

Think about a goal you set out to accomplish but did not complete. Focus on what you learned from trying to achieve the goal and share your experience in this journal entry. Usually, there is a sweet spot in every situation.

_____

_____

_____

_____

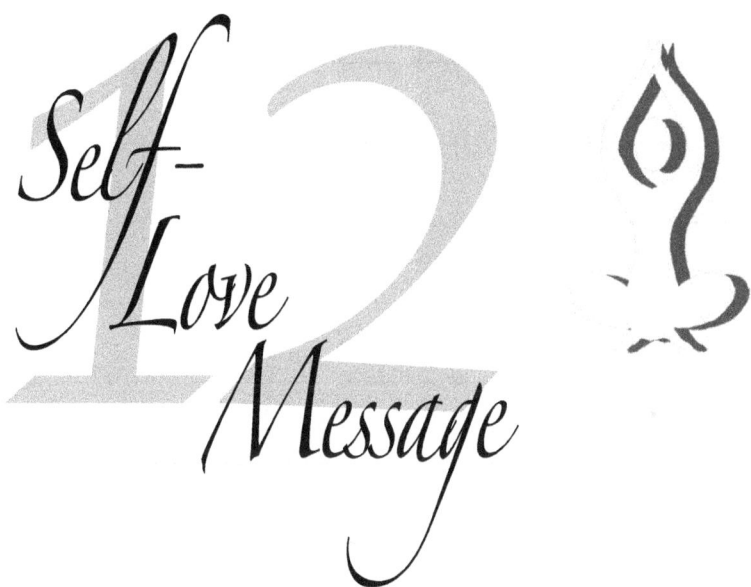

Self-Love Message

Sit quietly and breathe. Breathe without manipulating your breathing pattern and simply recognize your breath. Bring awareness to your heart and repeat this message mentally, *"I love myself, just as I am."* Sit quietly and repeat the message mentally. Take this with you throughout your day or evening.

Return to your journal and write your thoughts and feelings after repeating the centering thought throughout your day.

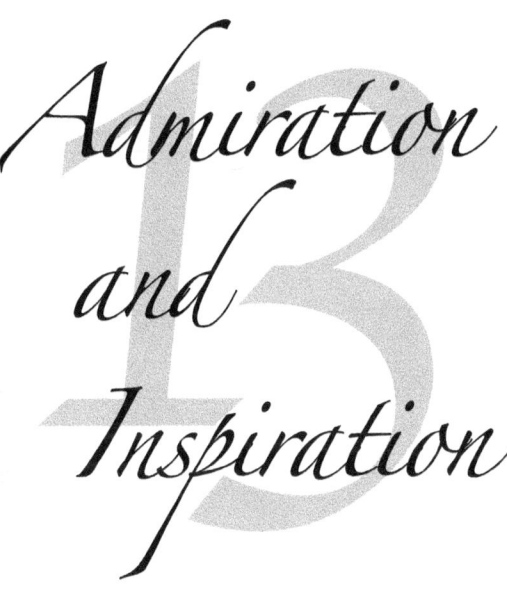
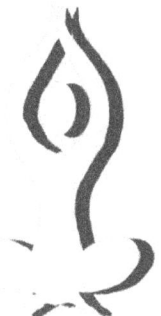

Admiration and Inspiration

"Do not be jealous of others' good qualities, but out of admiration, adopt them yourself." Buddha

Think about a person you admire. Please address what you admire about this person in his journal entry. Recognize and write about something you have in common and what qualities you can adopt.

_____

_____

_____

_____

14 Healthy Boundaries

Setting healthy boundaries will send your confidence to a new height. The capitulating effect of toxic relationships seems to happen all too often due to others' imposing beliefs. Attune to your feelings and notice what is no longer adequately serving you. Use your senses to help define your boundaries. Implement limits that are best for you without being attached to the outcome or concerned with being accepted by others.

This journal entry focuses on relationships and areas in your life where inserting a boundary for the sake of your personal growth is necessary. Journal your thoughts, boundary-setting goals, and plan to insert healthy limitations in relationships at home, work, and school.

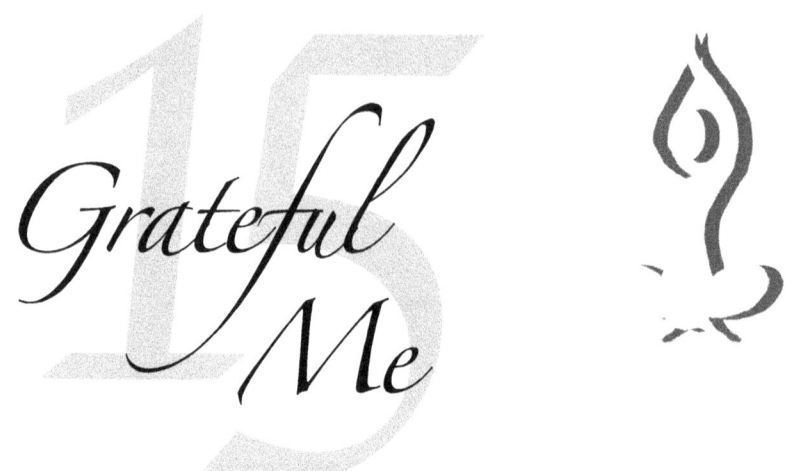

Grateful Me

"Be thankful for what you have; you'll end up having more. If you concentrate on what you don't have, you will never, ever have enough." -Oprah Winfrey

Write yourself a gratitude letter that describes what you're grateful for; commemorate the gifts you have received.

Dear _____

_____

_____

_____

_____

Self-Care is Essential

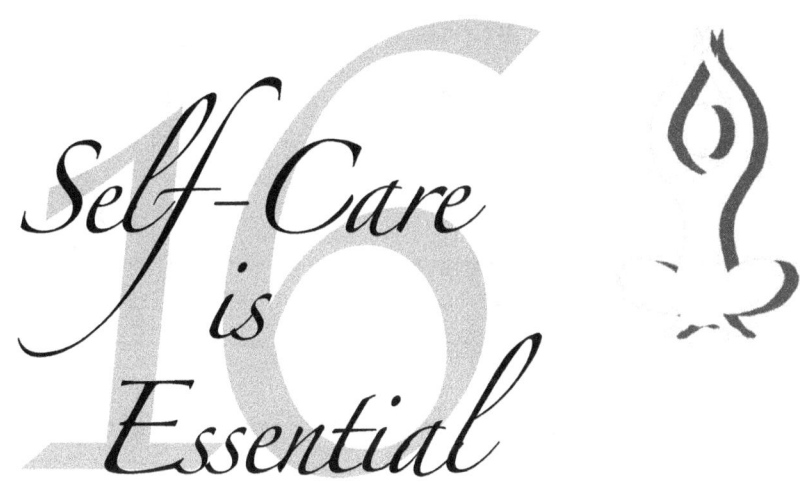

List three self-love activities you want to do and how you think they will benefit you. Journal the date that you will start and commit to positive change. Keep in mind that excuses get in the way of self-care.

Here are some self-care examples: Physical self-care possibly includes exercise or eating well. Emotional self-care may incorporate sitting with your feelings or doing something pleasurable. Spiritual self-care will be different from person to person but can be fulfilled through prayer, meditation, or church.

Mental health care can mean going to counseling, journaling, and healthy activities that are mentally stimulating.

17 Carefree Jubilee

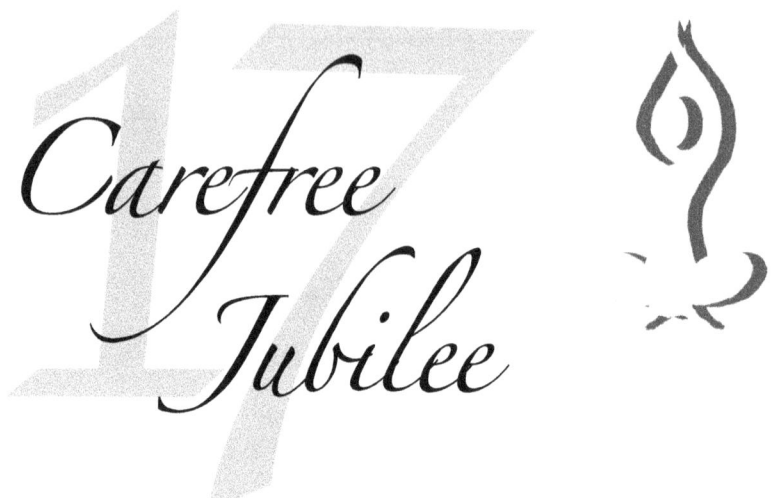

Visualize yourself in a peaceful and tranquil place. Take a moment and imagine what you will look like thirty years older than today-carefree and jubilee. Take note of your physical features. Describe your hair, skin, eyes, clothes, what you smell like, and feel like. What does the atmosphere around you look and feel like?

Now, return your focus to the older image of yourself. What message does the older and more seasoned version of yourself have for who you are today? Describe how you can apply the message to your life today— Journal your reflection of this visualization exercise.

Commit to Change 18

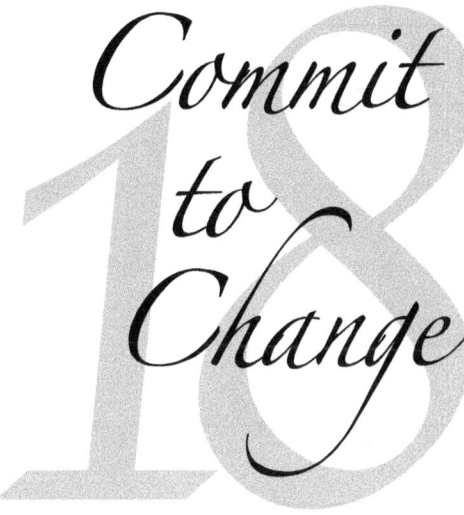
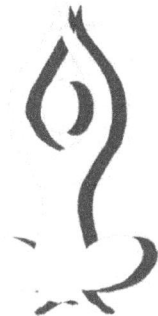

Commitment is like walking through a door of change for which you will never return. Identify one thing that you want to commit to and how the transformation will benefit your self-esteem. Identify the strengths that will help you start creating the difference and what strengths you will gain.

_____

_____

_____

_____

Significant Other

Think about your significant other and write about their likable characteristics and how they support you. If you do not have a significant other, think about who you want to attract. Write about how you imagine them to be. Note their characteristics and personality. Focus on how you can be the person you want to attract.

_____

_____

_____

_____

Motivating Mantra

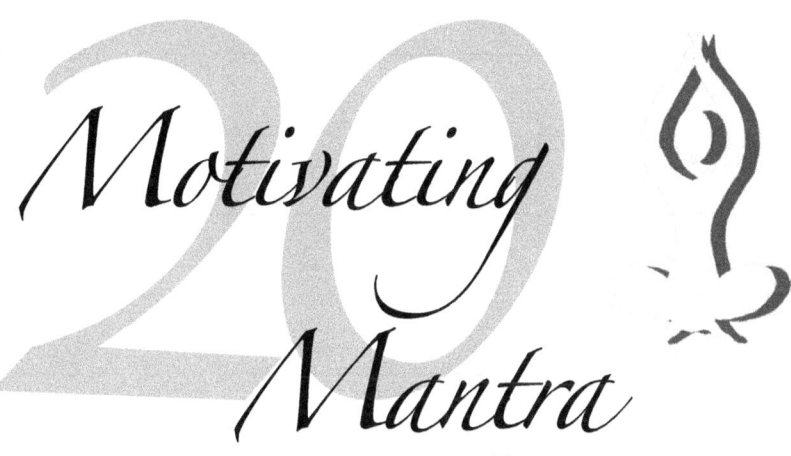

For this journaling prompt, set a timer for 5-10 minutes. Sit quietly and take some cleansing breaths and think of an intention. When you feel that your body is settled, think of a word that speaks to your purpose and use it as a motivating mantra (e.g., peace, acceptance, awareness, security, etc.) Journal your reflections about the meditation practice and note how your intuitive grasp applies to your reality.

_____

_____

_____

21 Me First

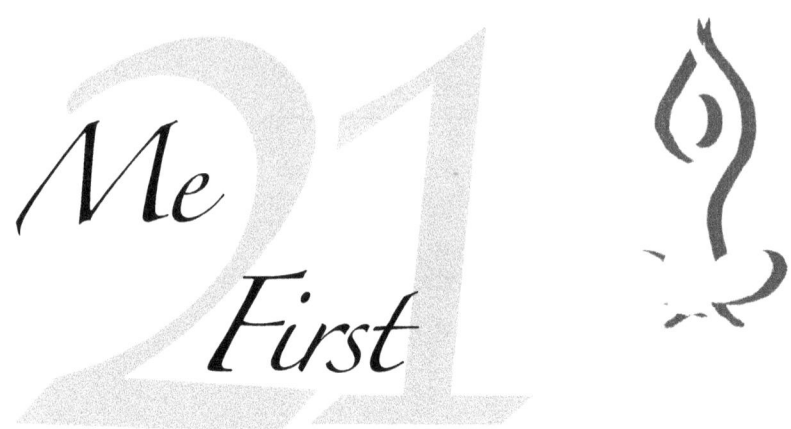

Most of us have heard the statement, "Take care of yourself before you take care of others." Caring for yourself first ensures that you remain mentally sound and physically healthy. Create a plan by identifying your self-care activities and a time to engage them. At least tune into the following three pillars of self-care- sufficient sleep, healthy diet, and exercise. After you have completed your activity, return to this journal entry to document your reflections. What inner awareness do you feel when engaging in self-care? How does self-care improve your self-esteem?

Personal Growth

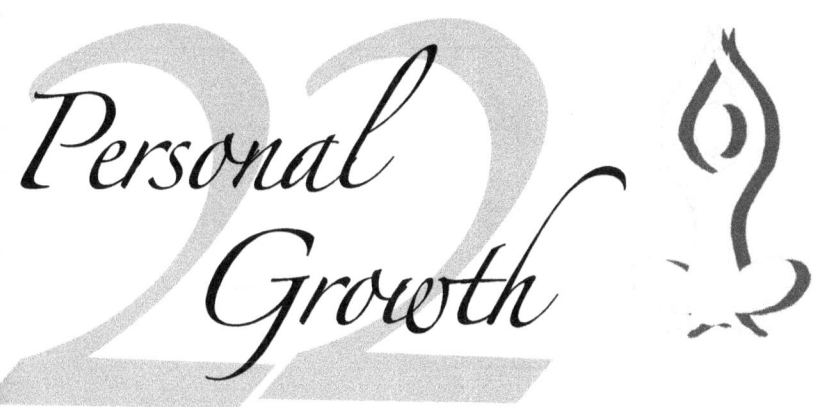

"You could not step twice into the same rivers; for other waters are ever flowing on to you."
-Heraclitus

Change happens in every moment- out with the old and in with the new. The choices you make today will create who you are tomorrow. Renew yourself. Observe the choices you make today. Recognize your personal growth and journal about your changes and progressions.

Practice 23 Silence

Have you ever tried to spend time in silence? Try spending a few hours or, better yet, one whole day in solitude. Your seclusion may include time away from friends and family, time away from television and social media. The only voice you will experience is your own. You will probably notice a tug-of-war in your mind. The frequency of fantasizing about the future and reminiscing on the past becomes heightened. You'll want to resist the 'monkey mind' and focus on the present. Stay in the 'Here and Now' during this exercise— describe how the practice of silence develops your self-esteem.

Accomplishments

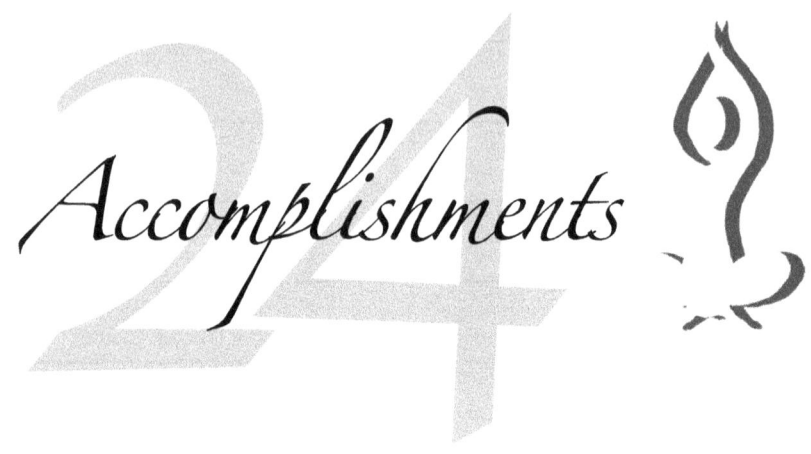

Write your top five achievements. Then, please choose the one you feel you learned the most from and journal about your new or renewed awareness because of your accomplishment.

1. _____
2. _____
3. _____
4. _____
5. _____

Letter of Recommendation

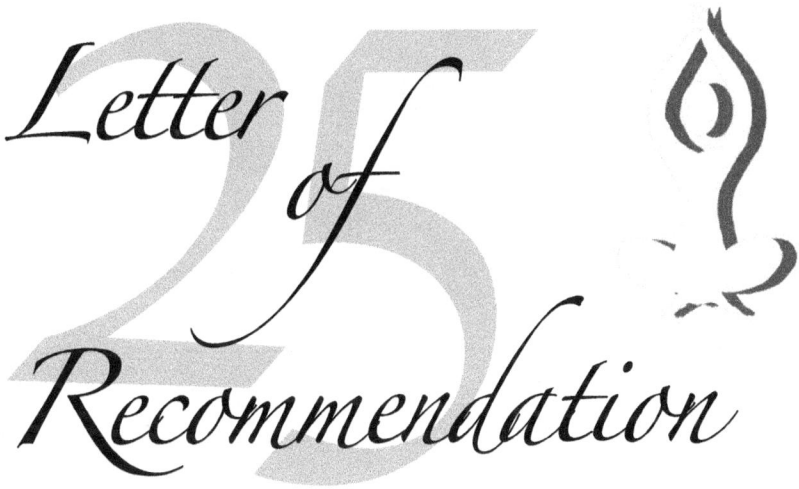

Imagine that you have to submit a reference of character letter for someone close to you. You would list all the excellent characteristics of this person. Write a reference letter for yourself with the same passion that you would write for that particular person. Return to this letter anytime you need a reminder of your character.

_____

_____

_____

_____

Self-Motivation

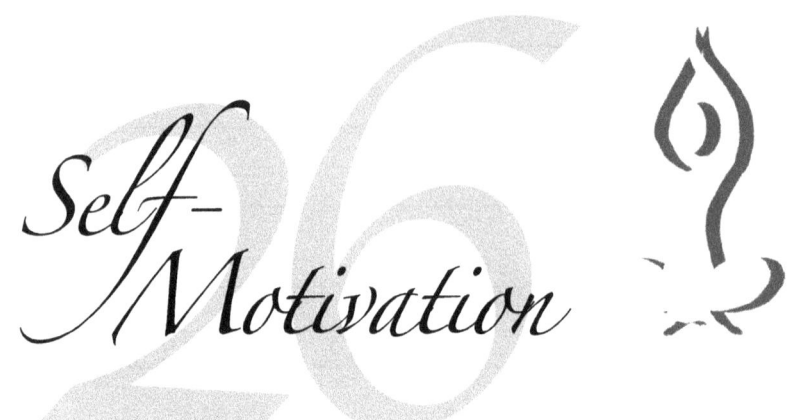

All development comes from motivation. To prepare for this journal entry, focus your attention on your heart's center. Describe the mental process you will use to motivate yourself. For example, the thought process might include reminiscing on the positive feelings gained from engaging in self-care, positive affirmations, or meditation.

"I promise to hold myself in positive regard routinely."

Remember, every time you honor yourself, you are one step closer to secured self-esteem. How will you motivate yourself on your journey of developing your esteem?

27 Who Am I?

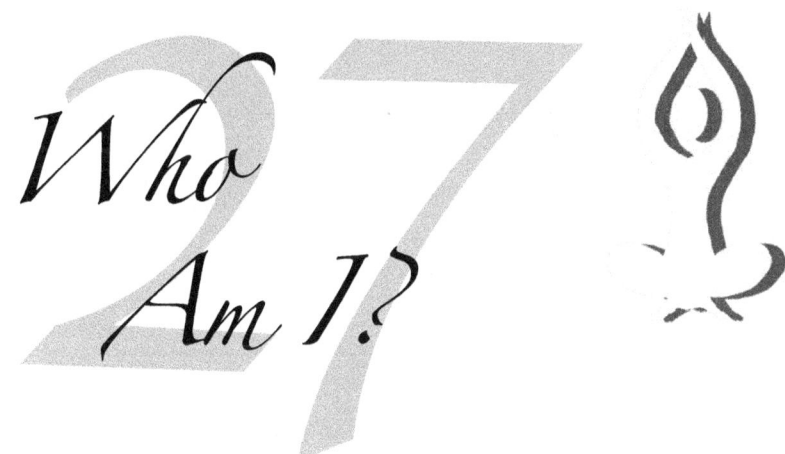

The purpose of the writing prompts for the next three days is to define your dreams and desires clearly. Follow the prompts and remember, designate a quiet space of solitude, meditate, and be truthful to yourself.

Write down all of the gifts that your creator has given you. Are you a lover, friend, musician, husband, wife, mother, teacher, business owner, CEO, sister, brother, a butterfly pollinating every delectable flower you see, or a spiritual being having a human experience? Who are you?

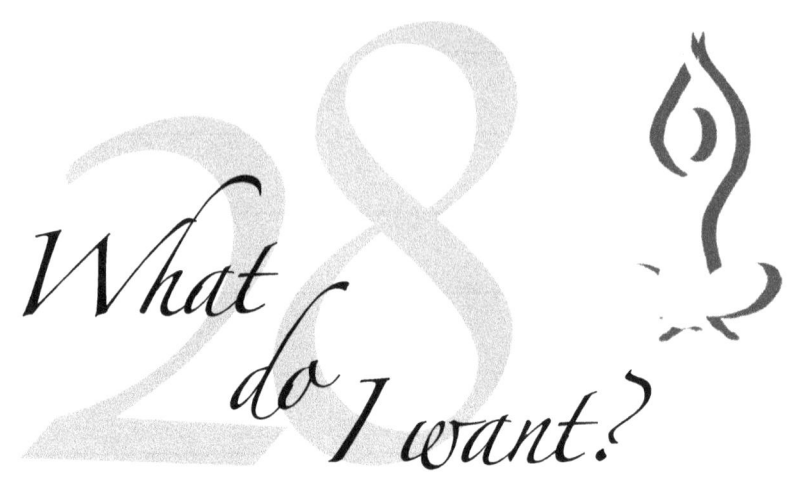

What do I want? 28

Here's your chance. If you have never visualized, focused, or sensed what you want, here's your chance. If the world was your oyster and you could have things your way, define it. Do you want a healthy mind and body, stop world hunger, material abundance, gain healthy friends, a spiritual awakening, personal growth? Do you want to set healthy boundaries, buy a new house, or live a life that you do not have to take a vacation from? Desires happen, first in mind and manifest in the physical. What do you want?

The Gift I Give

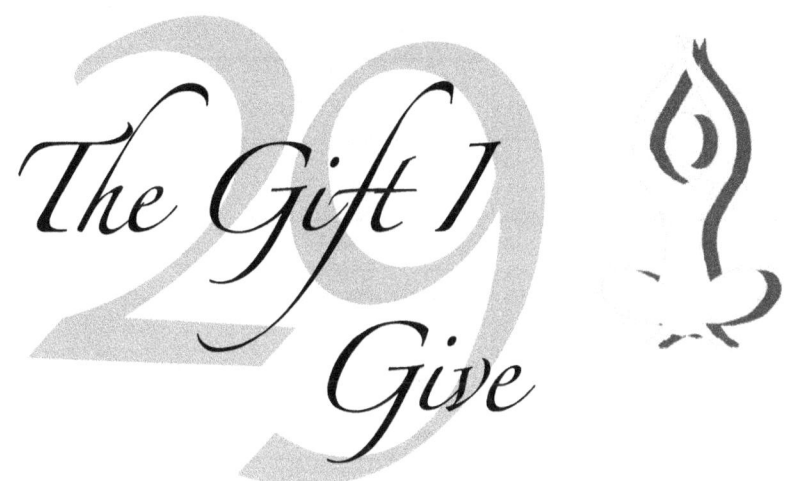

We live in a world of giving and receiving. Our breath, money flow, the cycle of water comes *in* and goes *out*. Ask yourself, "How can I serve?" You have defined who you are and what you want. Now, with all of your gifts, how do you share? Do you give back by volunteering, helping others, gardening, and giving food away, by becoming an attorney, counselor, fisherman, or that person on the corner giving lovely smiles to the passersby? How can you serve?

Completion

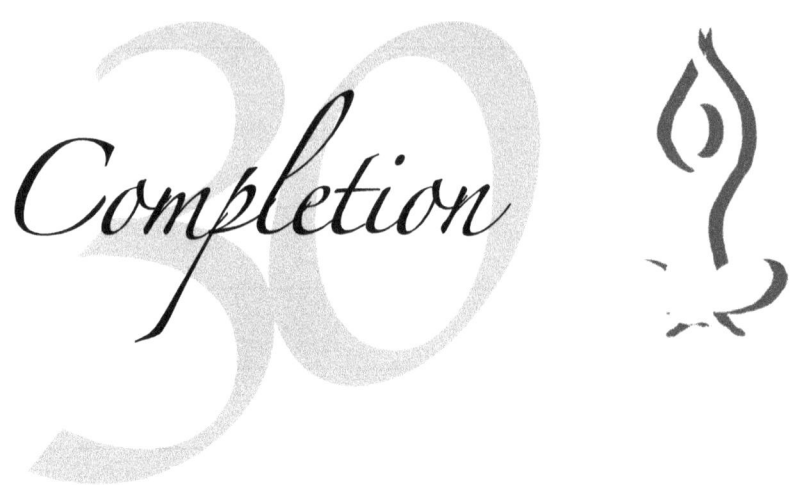

Congratulations, you have reached day 30!

On this 30th day of your self-esteem journaling journey, how do you feel about yourself? In this final entry, write about your progress. Describe how you felt about yourself 30 days ago and how you feel about yourself today. Revisit your chronicles when you need a reminder and a boost in confidence. Now continue your new self-care activity and continue to journal.

www.ingramcontent.com/pod-product-compliance
Lightning Source LLC
Chambersburg PA
CBHW070310100426
42743CB00011B/2432